DELIVERY WITHOUT STRESS

A Higher Chance of Safely Delivering A Healthy Child

A Book By Divinefavour Onofuevure

CONTENTS

Copyright 3
INTRODUCTION 3
GOOD NEWS 1 3
GOOD NEWS II..3
GOOD NEWS III 3
GOOD NEWS IV

....3

GOOD NEWS V 3
GOOD NEWS VI 3
SCRIPTURES TO MEDITATE ON CONCERNING THE
FORMATION OF YOUR BABY 3
FEATURE I..3
FEATURE II...3
FEATURE III 3
FEATURE IV 3
FEATURE V 3
FEATURE VI 3
FEATURE VII..3
SALVATION PRAYER..3
FINAL NOTE 3
TESTIMONY 3
About The Author..3
Books By This Author 3
Title Page 1

INTRODUCTION

The only prayer that is accepted by God is the one done according to his will and his will is his word.

The scripture says "And this is the confidence that we have in him, that if we ask anything according to his will he heareth us'' (1 John 5:14). "If ye abide in me and my words abide in you, ye shall ask whatever ye will and it shall be done unto you" (John 15:7).

It is important to know that God has provided for every area of our lives. He left nothing out including children and child birth. It is written in the Bible that we are covenant people and Christ has redeemed us from the curse of the law (Galatians 3:13) so we should continue to look into God's word for all he has provided for us in that redemption.

In the area of having babies, there have certainly been many things said over the years, some good and some bad, some right and some wrong. Most things we hear are from someone's experience and it was usually bad.

It is good news for us to know that God has wonderful promises for child bearing. You can change those negative testimonies and experience by knowing what God says concerning childbearing and delivery. Once you lay hold on God's word, and you begin to meditate on it, pray with the words and declare the words, I assure you no devil in the word will be able to stand against God's word, just try it.

Friends, enough of empty prayers without Gods word. This book is written to help you lay hold on the right scriptures for child birth and as you make use of it in prayer, I see you delivering your baby without stress. God's word cannot return to him void, it must accomplish the purpose which it has been sent. (Isaiah 55:11).

GOOD NEWS 1

But women will be saved through child bearing if they continue in faith, love, and holiness with propriety (I Timothy 2:15).

PRAYER AND CONFESSION

Lord, I thank you for your word; I believe I shall be saved throughout this pregnancy in Jesus name.

I reject every negative ministration of the devil and I cancel every spirit of death hanging around me in this pregnancy in Jesus name. I take cover under the blood of Jesus Christ.

GOOD NEWS II

The Hebrew women are very strong. They have their babies so quickly that we cannot get there in time. They are not slow in giving birth like Egyptian women (Exodus 1; 19-NLT).

PRAYER AND CONFESSION

Lord I thank you for making me strong in this pregnancy. I declare that I shall give birth quickly just like your word says.

I stand against every form of weakness in my body in Jesus Name. I reject any kind of prolonged labour; my labour shall be short in Jesus name.

GOOD NEWS III

Before she goes into labour she gives birth, before the pains come upon her, she delivers a son … yet no sooner is Zion in labour than she gives birth to her children.

Do I bring to the moment of birth and not give delivery? Says the Lord. Do I close up the womb when I bring to delivery? Says God (Isaiah 66:7-10 NIV).

PRAYER AND CONFESSION

Lord, I thank you for your word, I pray that I shall not have an unusual labour pains.

I pray that as you bring me to the moment of birth. You shall also help me to deliver my baby.

Therefore, I reject any kind of complication during my delivery period in Jesus name.

GOOD NEWS IV

They shall not labour in vain or bring forth (children) for sudden terror or calamity: for they shall be the descendants of the blessed of the Lord, and their offspring with them. (Isaiah 65:23, Amplified Bible)

PRAYER AND CONFESSION

Lord I agree and believe your word I decree that I shall never labour in vain. I will not have miscarriage. My baby will not be a still birth, I will never deliver a child that is deformed or disfigured. I shall come out healthy and my baby too healthy in Jesus name.

GOOD NEWS V

The Angel of the Lord encamps around those who fear him and he delivers them (psalm34:7).

PRAYER AND CONFESSION

Thank you Lord for giving your angels charge over me. I pray that your angels will surround me throughout this pregnancy and also during delivery period.

They shall deliver me and guard me against any kind of evil in Jesus name.

GOOD NEWS VI

Do not fear, for I am with you, do not be dismayed for I am your God I will strengthen you and help you I will uphold you with my righteous hand (Isaiah 41:10).

PRAYER AND CONFESSION

Father I come before you in the mighty name of Jesus and in the covenant of blood. I rebuke fear, doubt and unbelief. I trust in the Lord.

I will not fear or doubt the promises of God concerning me in this pregnancy.

I refuse to let my heart be troubled or afraid no matter what I hear or see in this pregnancy for I know you are with me in Jesus name.

SCRIPTURES TO MEDITATE ON CONCERNING THE FORMATION OF YOUR BABY

Psalm 139 vs. 13 (NIV)

For you created my inmost being; you knit me together in my mother's womb.

Isaiah 44 vs. 12 (NIV)

This is what the Lord says he who made you, who formed you in the womb, and he will help you.

Galatians 1 vs. 15 (NIV)

But when God, who set me apart from my mother's womb and called me by his grace, was pleased...'

Note: these scriptures show that it is the Lord that formed your baby in the womb. Your baby can hear the word of God even right there in the womb, because their spirit is alive and alert. Use these scriptures to speak over the baby's life and features.

FEATURE I

BABY'S SPIRIT

"For he shall be great in the sight of the lord and he shall drink neither wine nor strong drink and he shall be filled with the Holy ghost even from his mother's womb" (luke1vs.15).

PRAYER AND DECLARATION

Father I thank you for your word. Baby I declare that you will be tender towards God and the things of God. You will be saved at an early age and be filled with the spirit of God on   time.

FEATURE II

HEART

"I will give you a new heart and put a new spirit within you; I will take the heart of stone out of your flesh and give you a heart of flesh" (Ezekiel 36vs.26).

"Let not your heart be troubled; ye believe in God, believe also in me. (John14vs.1).

PRAYER AND DECLARATION

Father I declare over my baby's heart that it will be strong, and healthy and untroubled. There shall be no complication. It is functioning properly in Jesus name.

FEATURE III

BABY'S TEMPERAMENT

And beside this, giving all diligence, add to your faith virtue, and to virtue knowledge, and to knowledge temperance and to temperance patience and to temperance patience and to patience godliness, to godliness brotherly kindliness, and to brotherly kindness charity.

PRAYER AND DECLARATION

Father I pray and declare over my baby's temperance to be calm and full of peace. Baby, you will not be easily angry or irritated, you will be a joyful baby all the days of your life.

FEATURE IV

BONES

He keepeth all his bone, not one of them is broken (Psalm34vs.20).

PRAYER AND DECLARATION

Father I speak to my baby's bone to be strong, healthy, straight and none shall be broken in Jesus name.

FEATURE V

BLOOD

'And when I passed by thee, and saw the polluted in thine own blood, I said unto thee when thou wast in thy blood, live; yea I said unto thee when thou was in thy blood, live' (Ezekiel16vs.6).

PRAYER AND DECLARATION

Father I declare over my baby's blood to be normal, healthy. Maintain proper blood sugar, no pollution in the blood. The blood of Jesus is flowing together with my baby's blood in Jesus name.

FEATURE VI

TEETH, HAIR, LIPS, EYE, NECK.

"How beautiful you are, my love! How your eye shine with love behind your veil. Your hair dances, like a flock of goats bounding down the hills of Gilead. Your teeth are as white as sheep that have just been shorn and washed. Not one of them is missing. They are all perfectly matched. Your lips are like a scarlet ribbon; how lovely they are when you speak. Your cheeks glow behind your veil. Your neck is like the tower of h David round and smooth (song of solomon4vs.1-4).

PRAYER AND DECLARATION

Father I speak to every part of my baby's body to function properly and fully developed as you intended. His ears hear perfectly, his eyes not dim, teeth strong, not prone to cavities, neck smooth, digestive and respiratory system function normally.

I declare health, wholeness, soundness, spirit, soul and body from the top of the head to the bottom of the feet. I speak to the cord to be in perfect position and length not around the baby's   neck.

FEATURE VII

SLEEPING HABITS

And the Lord God caused a deep sleep to fall upon Adam, and he slept (Genesis3vs.1).

PRAYER AND DECLARATION

Father, I declare that my baby shall always have deep sleep at night and allow me to sleep and rest, no restlessness and unusual crying at night .you give your beloved sleep in Jesus name.

SALVATION PRAYER

For the word of God to work effectively for you, you need to give your life to Jesus. Simply pray this prayer;

Heavenly father, I come to you in the name of Jesus, I pray and ask you to come into my heart and be Lord over my life.

According to Romans 10:9-10 "If thou shall confess with your mouth the Lord Jesus, and shall believe in your heart that God has raised him from the dead, you shall be saved" I do that now, I confess that Jesus is Lord, and believe in my heart that God raised him from the dead. I am now born again! I am a child of Almighty God! I am saved.

FINAL NOTE

Now! You are born again; believe every word written in this book concerning your delivery. I see you delivering without stress in Jesus name. You will deliver successfully and you shall carry your baby in your arms for that is God's plan and will for you. Remain blessed.

For more information contact:

Divinefavour Onofuevure

Living Faith Church, Ughelli

End of Osadjere Estate,

Off Isoko Road,

Ughelli Delta State

Nigeria.

Phone-Number: +2347043301090

Facebook: DivineFavour Onofuevure

Email: divinefavouronofuevure@gmail.com

TESTIMONY

I DELIVERED MY BABY SAFE AND SOUND WITHOUT STRESS BUT THE DEVIL REFUSED TO GIVE UP, THE FOLLOWING DAY AS THE NURSES WERE BATHING THE BABY, HE FELL DOWN FROM A NURSE HAND, IT WAS AS IF THE END OF MY BABY HAS COME BUT TO GOD BE THE GLORY AS I STARTED PRAYING, CONFESSING GOD'S WORD MY BABY'S HEALTH WAS RESTORED. NO DEFORMITY, NO SCAR,

MY BABY IS NOW A BIG BOY. GLORY BE TO GOD.

Chidalu Ibeneme .

USA

ABOUT THE AUTHOR

DivineFavour Onofuevure

DivineFavour Onofuevure is a prolific writer and author of Framing Your World, Foundation of Sapphires, Delivery without Stress and Kings Kids confession book (KKS). She is the Editor in Chief of Teens World Digest (Quarterly programme for teenagers in schools).
She is a graduate of University of Calabar, Cross River State with a Bachelor of Arts Degree in English and Literary Studies. She also has Masters in Public Administration (MPA) from University of Ilorin, Kwara State and PGD Education from National Teachers Institution (NTI). Also, a graduate of World of Faith Bible Institute (WOFBI) and Haggai Institute Alumni Association of Nigeria, Ilorin.
She is the CEO and governor of Teens World Harvesters Foundation. She has been a resource person in various seminars conducted by different secondary schools. She is presently teaching in Transcorp Power Limited Staff Schools, Ughelli, Delta State, Nigeria. She is a wife, mother and serves with her husband, Pastor Andrew, in Living Faith Church (Winners Chapel) Ughelli, Delta State, Nigeria.

BOOKS BY THIS AUTHOR

CREATING YOUR ACADEMIC WORLD

www.ingramcontent.com/pod-product-compliance
Lightning Source LLC
Chambersburg PA
CBHW060911260726
48661CB00008B/3586